MILKING YOUR GOATS

WHAT YOU NEED

TO KNOW GUIDE

Felicity McCullough

Paperback Edition

My Lap Shop Publishers

Plymouth, England

www.mylapshop.com

ISBN: 978-1-78165-047-9

Series: Goat Knowledge 10

Disclaimer

This book is meant to be STRICTLY AN EDUCATIONAL AND INFORMATIONAL TOOL ONLY. The suggestions contained in this material might not be suitable for everyone. It is not intended to provide diagnosis or treatment. The author obtained the information from sources believed to be reliable and from personal experience. Although the best effort was made by the author, there are no guarantees as to the accuracy or completeness of the contents within this work.

The author does not guarantee the accuracy of any information or content in resources or websites listed or cited within this work. Additionally, the author, publisher and distributors never give medical, legal, accounting or any other type of professional advice. The reader must always seek those services from competent professionals that can review the particular circumstances. Mention of any product, brand or website is NOT an endorsement or recommendation of that product, service or usage.

The medical field is a very dynamic field that is constantly undergoing research, modifications and advancements and therefore information contained in this book should always be researched further and A VETERINARIAN OR OTHER SPECIALIST SHOULD BE CONSULTED where appropriate.

Any and all application of the information contained in this book is of the sole responsibility of the person performing said action. The author, publisher and distributors particularly disclaim any liability, loss, or risk taken by individuals who directly or indirectly act on the information herein. All readers must accept full responsibility for their use of this material.

My Lap Shop Publishers

Plymouth, England

www.mylapshop.com

Acknowledgement

The publisher thanks Danielle Shurskis for her support and help in bringing these series of books and articles to publication.

Table of Contents

Why Goats?

Goat's milk is a delicious alternative to cow's milk. There are a number of myths and misconceptions about goat's milk, including that it has a strong smell and taste. If properly collected, stored and handled, this is not true. Goat's milk does have a unique and distinctive taste.

Raising goats for milk instead of cows offer a number of advantages. One of the most noteworthy advantages is that goats are roughly a sixth of the size of cows and eat a lot less. Consequently, they also produce a lot less manure and are easier to manage and handle. You also need less land to raise goats. On the other hand, this also means that they produce less milk. They produce approximately five times less milk than cows.

Goats are slightly more efficient than cows in terms of converting feed to milk. This means that they are able to make slightly more milk out of one pound of feed, for example, than a cow is capable of. According to Oklahoma Cooperative

Extension Service, on average it takes roughly 70 pounds of rations to produce one more gallon of milk.

Goats also tend to have a slightly longer productive life. Whereas cows normally produce milk from four to six years, goats can produce from eight to ten years. This means that you will need to replace goats less often than cows.

There are a few challenges related to raising goats. One is that they are seasonal breeders. Being a seasonal breeder means that they breed during the fall and winter and kid in the spring, making it more difficult to have milk all year. Goats also tend to require more work than cows, resulting in a higher labour cost per gallon. The labour cost per gallon is approximately double for goat's milk.

Milk Composition and Comparison

Anyone who has tasted goat's milk knows that it is very distinctive and unique. It is actually very similar to cow's milk in terms of composition, with some important differences.

Goat's milk is made mostly of water with a little protein, fat, calcium, vitamins and milk sugars. Goat's milk is made up of roughly: 87% water, 4.25% fat, 3.52% protein, 4.27% lactose, 0.86% Ash and 8.75% non-fat solids (Oklahoma Cooperative Extension Service).

Water

Roughly 87% of milk is water, whether it is goat, cow, or even human milk. Sheep milk contains slightly less water, around 81%. This is one of the reasons why does producing milk needs to be provided with as much fresh, clean water as she can drink.

Protein

There is around 3.52% protein in goat's milk. There is a structural difference between the protein found in goat's milk and the protein found in cow's milk. It is now suggested that this fact is why people who are allergic to cow's milk can drink goat's milk.

Protein is responsible for the curd made when making cheeses. Curd made from goat's milk is softer than that of cow's milk, making it dissolve more quickly, thus making it more digestible.

Fat

Lipids or fat contained in goat milk can vary greatly, from 3% to 6%. According to the UC Davis site, goat's milk contains 11 to 25 mg per 100 grams of cholesterol.

A great many factors affect the amount of fat in the milk. Among these factors are genetics or breed, the quality and quantity of feed, season, and stage of lactation just to name a few factors. One of the only major differences between goat and cow milk is that goat's milk has a different amount of specific short chain fatty acids, namely capric, caprylic and caproic acids. These are what give goat's milk its unique taste.

Goat's milk is said to be naturally homogenized with smaller fat globules than that of cow's milk. It is often claimed that goat's milk is more digestible than cow's milk, because of the size of the fat globules. These claims are currently under investigation and subject to research.

Carbohydrates

The major carbohydrate found in goat's milk is sugar, specifically lactose.

Vitamins

Goat's milk, similarly to cow's milk, is very rich in vitamins. Normally, the most abundant vitamins are vitamin A, D and choline, which is a B-complex vitamin. There is roughly double the amount of Vitamin A in goat's milk than cow's milk. There are also trace amounts of Ascorbic acid/C, Biotin/B7, Folic Acid/B9, Nicotinic Acid/B3, Riboflavin/B2, Thiamine/B1, Vitamin B12, and Vitamin B6.

Minerals

As most people are aware, the most abundant mineral in milk is calcium. This is true of both goat's and cow's milk.

Goat's milk generally has more calcium, phosphorus, chlorine, magnesium and potassium than cow's milk.

Lactation

Lactation begins with the birth of the offspring and usually lasts about ten months in dairy goats.

Amounts Produced

Goats do not produce as much as dairy cows. A goat can produce anywhere from six to eight pounds a day. How much milk is produced depends on many factors, including the quantity and quality of her diet as well as genetics, which is associated to breed.

Nutritional Demands

It is a very demanding period in the female's production cycle, because there is a huge metabolic change during a time when there is also usually a negative energy balance. The doe is in negative energy balance, because the energy levels are very high and it is physically impossible for the doe to eat enough to fulfil her nutritional requirements.

Her nutritional requirements are especially high because it takes a lot of nutrients and energy to produce milk and although the rumen capacity is increasing, there is physically not enough room for the amount of forage she needs. During lactation, the most important nutrient is energy, because it is the most likely to be deficient.

Extra nutrition is needed to prevent Pregnancy Toxaemia and Milk Fever, two disorders that result from a lack of nutrients. Pregnancy Toxaemia is caused by a lack of energy. Milk Fever is caused by a lack of calcium. Milk Fever usually appears one to three weeks after kidding.

Nutrient requirements vary by species, age, size and number of young. Forage is not enough, even high-energy forage, because there is not enough space in the rumen to fit the amount needed per day. You will have to supplement grain.

Remember to make any and all dietary changes slowly to avoid Overeating Disease. Overeating disease is a condition caused by abrupt dietary changes, which result in the death of populations of microbes and the proliferation of pathological microbes.

The best thing to do is to balance your ration for your does. You can find websites where this can be done online, or download programs, or files to help with this, though this is not what most people do. Most people tend to use a rule of thumb instead.

Do not forget your water supply as well. Lactating does require roughly 100% more water than non-lactating does. The water needs to be fresh, clean and with an appropriate temperature, meaning that you will need heated containers in places where the water freezes in winter. If you do not heat the water, the does will not drink and their milk production will fall. Also remember to clean the containers every day.

Common Rules of Thumb for Nutrition

When talking about how much feed an animal needs, there are some terms that are used that may be confusing. Usually the amount of feed recommended will be given as dry matter intake or DMI, instead of giving measurements in pounds of feed. The plants that are the main part of the ruminant diet are made up mostly of water. Everything else is dry matter, including the fat, protein, and carbohydrates etcetera. This can often make calculating diets tricky.

TDN is another measurement that you will probably come across when researching ruminant diets. TDN stands for Total Digestible Nutrients.

According to Jeff Semler in a Ewe and Doe Management Series Webinar, a doe with a single baby should ingest around 3.6% of its bodyweight in dry matter intake, 65% TDN, 13.5% crude protein, 0.32% calcium and 0.26% phosphorus. A doe with twins needs 4% of her bodyweight in DMI, 65% TDN, 15% crude protein, 0.39% calcium and 0.29% phosphorus.

It is advisable to give does a free-choice of good alfalfa hay, with roughly one pound of grain for every 2 quarts of milk produced, as well as free access to a mineral mix. Diet can be supplemented with fruits and vegetables if desired, although if selling milk be aware that some foods can taint the milk, such as bananas and wild garlic.

Alfalfa hay is high in calcium. Calcium can also be supplemented in complete grain mixes, or in mineral supplements such as dicalcium phosphate, limestone and bone meal from poultry. It is illegal in most countries, to give any supplement to ruminants made from ruminants.

Drying the Doe

Eventually the doe will need to be "dried". This means that she will stop producing milk for a time in order to let the tissues that make up the udder rest and recuperate. The animal cannot produce milk continuously.

This naturally happens when the kids are weaned or you can induce drying. Start reducing the grain given to the does one or two weeks prior to the weaning date. Cut the grain completely on the week that the kids are to be weaned. Also change to lower quality grass hay, or even straw during the last few days, right before weaning and continue until the udders have dried. Keep giving water.

Milking Your Goats

Be sure to test your animals annually for TB and Brucellosis.

Equipment Preparation

If you use a wash cloth to clean the udders, you will need to sterilize it in boiling water. Add cool water until you obtain a hot, yet comfortable temperature. Make sure that your jug and milking can is clean and dry. Prepare your sterile filtering cloth and lid.

Doe Preparation

Bring the goat to the stanchion and secure her head. Put a feed bucket with her grain for the day. Use the hot wash cloth to wash the udder and teats, removing hair and dust. This process also stimulates the let-down of the milk. Wring out the cloth and use it to dry the udder.

Milk the Doe

Begin milking. Discard the first squeezes, because bacteria from the environment will be near the teat opening. Place the milking can on a "milking board". A "milking board" is a small piece of wood that keeps the milking can above the surface where the goat steps. This is not a requirement.

When it comes time to actually milk the goat, you have a few options. You can manually milk, or you can use a machine. There are a few manual devices which can help, or you can purchase whole dairy machine systems.

To manually milk, pinch the top of the teat with your index and thumb in order to prevent milk from rising and then use the other fingers to squeeze the rest of the teat. Then release the teat. Repeat until no more milk is removed from squeezing the teat. Then massage the udder vigorously yet gently, so as not to hurt the doe and squeeze a few more times.

Record Data

If you keep records, which is advisable, then you should weigh the milk and record it now. Keeping records is advisable, because it gives you a way to keep track of how your animals are doing. It also helps with your business, by keeping track of expenses and whether your does are "paying for their keep". You will also be able to know when it is time to cull, meaning selling a doe. Does that repeatedly get sick, or abort their offspring are examples of animals which should be culled.

Filter the Milk

Pour the milk through a sterile fine-weave cloth to remove dust and hair. Sterilize this cloth by boiling and then completely drying.

Cleaning Up the Area

Release the goat and put her back with the others. Then, sweep the area including the stanchion and the "milking board". Next, wash everything and dry with a wrung out cloth.

Chill the Milk

One of the most important steps in making sure that your milk has the longest shelf-life possible is to rapidly cool the milk down. Do this by putting the milk containers in a bigger container with cold water. You can put ice in the water as well. Also be sure to label the milk with the date. Never add warm milk to cool milk. You can mix older cooled milk with newer cooled milk. Milk should be good for at least a week without pasteurisation.

Cleaning Up the Equipment

After you put the milk to chill, rinse out the milking can. Then wash it with hot water and soap. Rinse well and let the can air dry. Boil the filtering cloth for a few minutes and let dry in the sun, if possible.

Pasteurization

Many people drink or sell their milk without pasteurizing it. This is fine if you are completely aware of the health status of your goats and if the milk was properly handled.

Pasteurization is the process where food is heated with the intent of reducing the population of microbes. Note that the intent is to *reduce* and *not* to destroy. This is not sterilization.

There are a few different types of pasteurization that goat milk can undergo:

Low Pasteurization

Low pasteurization is the process where the milk is heated to 74° C for 15 seconds. It doesn't alter the milk except to inactivate some enzymes.

High Pasteurization

High Pasteurization is the process where the milk is heated to 90° C for 15 seconds. This process inactivates most of the enzymes in the milk and makes some of the whey proteins insoluble.

Sterilization

Sterilization occurs when you heat the milk to 118º C for 20 seconds. This is not used because it alters the milk, turning it brownish and changing both protein and sugars. One form of sterilization, Ultra-High Temperature (UHT) is a process where milk is heated to 145º C for a few seconds, thus sterilizing the milk while minimizing chemical changes.

Tips on Management Practices

Now will be discussed a number of excellent management tips used to produce the highest quality milk.

Managing the Doe

We recommend separating your milk producing herd into lots, depending on the doe's age and the amount of young, if possible.

Doelings are young does that are gestating or producing milk for the first time. They are around one year old. Separating these doelings is important, because doelings tend to be pushed around by the older does and do not receive as much feed. They require more feed because not only are they producing milk or a foetus, they are still growing.

The more offspring that a doe produces means that the teats are stimulated more, resulting in more milk production.

A higher production of milk means a higher nutritional requirement. So, does with triplets need more feed than does with twins and these does need more than does with a single baby.

If you combine all of these animals in one herd, there will be some animals getting more feed than needed, with consequent weight gain and others that are not getting enough, with consequent diminishing of milk production.

We do understand that creating several lots is not viable in operations with a small herd of animals. If possible, try separating at feeding time.

It is important, no matter the operation to keep an eye on body condition and to adjust feed as needed. In other words, if the females are losing weight, give more feed and if they are gaining weight, give less. Always remember to make dietary changes gradual.

Another management practice that is often used is to de-worm all the does right before they kid. A modified management technique is to evaluate using the FEMACHA System©, or the Five Point Check system© and de-worm the does that show signs of a rise in worm population instead of simply de-worming the whole herd.

People do this due to something called the Periparturient Egg Rise. This phenomenon describes a temporary loss of immunity in the doe right around the time of kidding, resulting in a rise in the population of worms. Using the evaluation systems is done to avoid developing drug resistance in the worm populations for as long as possible.

A word of caution is needed regarding the de-wormer Valbazen®. This drug should not be used in the first 30 days of pregnancy.

Managing the Feeders

Make sure that all the does in the herd can eat at the same time. If there is only room for a percentage of the herd, the submissive does will always lose out to the dominant females and will end up losing weight, while the dominants ones gain weight.

Managing the Milk

People have often complained that goat's milk has a very unpleasant odour or taste. This is not true if the milk is properly manipulated, collected and stored. The secret is hygiene. Goat's milk can be kept as fresh as cow's milk for as long as cow's milk as well.

Bucks are the male goats and they do have a very distinctive and unpleasant odour during mating season due to the fact that they spray themselves with urine. Bucks should always be kept separately and not be anywhere near where the does are milked. Keep at least 50 feet between bucks and the milking station.

Keep your does healthy. Illnesses or diseases will affect the quality of your milk. All your animals should look healthy and alert with no physical signs of illness. This includes mastitis, or the inflammation of the teats, which will be discussed in greater detail in the section entitled Mastitis below. If necessary, send a small sample of your milk to a laboratory for testing. You should test especially for Brucellosis and Tuberculosis in your herd once a year.

Milk is easily affected by the environment. In other words, make sure that the place where you milk is free of any strong odours. Also make sure that the area is well ventilated, clean and dry. Bacteria love a damp area to grow.

Keep goats clean as well. The does' udders should be clipped and cleaned with mild soap and water and disinfected before each milking. Also make sure that all equipment that comes in direct contact with the milk is cleaned regularly and properly disinfected, including the milker's hands and arms.

Get the milk cooled and refrigerated as soon as possible after milking. Cooling the temperature will prevent the growth of bacteria. Store it in seamless aluminium, stainless steel, or glass containers. Containers made from copper, plastic and tin can cause off-tastes in the milk.

Mastitis

The one disease that causes the most problems with milk is Mastitis, or the inflammation of the mammary gland, commonly known as the udder.

Forms of Mastitis

There are two forms of mastitis, subclinical and clinical. Clinical mastitis is the classic form where the udders are showing that they are infected and altered. Alterations can include pain, feeling hot to the touch and becoming swollen.

Milk is also altered. Milk can present with clots, flakes, and discolouration, or become watery. Depending on the severity of the infection, systemic symptoms such as fever, depression and weakness may also be present.

Subclinical mastitis is the form where the goat seems healthy and normal, yet there is an infection in the udder. Subclinical mastitis is a problem because it is more prevalent, yet harder to detect.

Subclinical mastitis alters the taste of the milk and decreases the amount of milk produced. This form of mastitis also raises the amount of somatic cells in the milk, which is detectable in milk tests.

Common Causes of Mastitis

There are a few different species of microorganisms that can cause mastitis. The most important species is *Staphylococcus aureus.* Three other important species are *Streptococcus spp., Pasteurella haemolytica* and

Corynebacterium pseudotuberculosis.

There are actually three different species of Streptococcus that are important, namely *S. agalactia*, *S. uberis* and *S. dysgalactia*. Coliforms and *Mycoplasma spp.* are less common, but can also cause mastitis.

Treating Mastitis

Treating mastitis involves both a change in management and the administration of some medications. There are products available on the market for intramammary application, meaning that it is applied into the affected teat. You may also need to administer systemic antibiotics, such as Penicillin, Erythromycin, or Tetracycline. Severe cases may also require antihistamines, anti-inflammatory agents and even fluid therapy.

What to Do with the Milk

Now that you've obtained the milk and it is chilled and stored to perfection, what will you do with it? The answer to this question depends on why you are milking goats.

If you simply want to provide your family with fresh milk to drink, you are all set. If, on the other hand, you are looking to make a profit from your dairy business, then you are probably interested in selling.

There are a number of options available to the seller.

The easiest and perhaps most profitable is to simply sell the milk. You do not need to process the milk in this case, simply chill it.

You will need to check the laws in your area if you want to sell it raw. Some countries require milk to be pasteurized to be sold commercially.

Goat's milk can be processed into anything that cow's milk is used for. Cheeses and yoghurts are the most common, yet evaporated milk and dried milk products are also possibilities.

Yoghurt is made also with a culture or a starter added to the goat's milk. Goat's milk makes even more palatable yoghurt than cow's milk, because it is less acidic and has less lactose.

There are a number of cheeses that are made with goat's milk, including a type of cottage cheese, a baker's cheese, cream cheese, Neufchatel, Domiati cheese, and Feta cheese.

The basic cheese process is to take the milk, add bacteria and coagulate the protein. Then the curd is recovered and treated. Some cheeses are then sold. Others are aged first.

Resources

Semler, Jeff. Lactation. 2011
Ewe and Doe Management
Series. Available at: -
https://connect.moo.umd.edu/p4
2131942/.

The Dairy Research &
Information Center (DRINC).
Dairy Goat Milk Composition.
Available at: -
http://drinc.ucdavis.edu/goat1.ht
m.

Richardson, Curtis W. Let's
Compare Dairy Goats and Cows.
Oklahoma State University.

Available at: -
http://oklahoma4h.okstate.edu/lit
ol/file/animal/dairy/N-
424_web.pdf.

Fankhauser, David B. Handling
of Fresh Raw Milk. 2000.
Available at:

http://biology.clc.uc.edu/fankhaus
er/cheese/milkhandling.htm.

Copyright 2012 ©

My Lap Shop Publishers

Unit 222, Plymouth, Devon PL1 1SB UK

Publishers

My Lap Shop Publishers

91 Mayflower Street, Unit 222,

Plymouth, Devon, PL1 1SB

United Kingdom

Tel: +44 (0)871 560 5297

www.mylapshop.com

www.goatlapshop.com

First Edition September 2012

ISBN - 978-1-78165-047-9

About Felicity McCullough

Felicity McCullough has written several books about preventative health care for goats.

The website dedicated to goats www.goatlapshop.com has a wide variety of topics and resources that relate to goats, including the Charlie And Isabella's Magical Adventures Series of Children's Books, suitable for bed-time reading that are beautifully illustrated.

Goat Knowledge Series Titles

How To Keep Goats Healthy #1
ISBN: 978-1-78165-021-9
Golden Guernsey Goats #2
ISBN: 978-1-78165-022-6
A Simple Guide To The Goat's
Digestive System #3
ISBN: 978-1-78165-024-0
Success Guide For Raising
Healthy Goats #4
ISBN: 978-1-78165-026-4
Managing Goat Nutrition: What
You Need To Know A Simple
Guide #5
ISBN: 978-1-78165-027-1
Plants And Goats An Easy To
Read Guide #6
ISBN: 978-1-78165-038-7
Goat Housing, Bedding, Fencing,
Exercise Yards And Pasture
Management Guide #7
ISBN: 978-1-78165-040-0
Weaning Your Goat Kids A
Simple Guide #8

ISBN: 978-1-78165-042-4
How To Breed Goats And
Manage Gestation A Simple For
Guide #9
ISBN: 978-1-78165-045-5

Other Goat Books and Articles

By Felicity McCullough

www.goatlapshop.com

Boar Goats
Charlie And Isabella's Magical
Adventure
Charlie And Isabella Meet Jacob
Charlie And Isabella's Second
Adventure With Jacob
Charlie And Isabella's Magical
Adventures Compendium
Diseases of Goats
Goat Basics

Goat Breed: Golden Guernsey Goats
Goat Videos
How To Keep Goats Healthy
Nigerian Dwarf Goats
Nimbkar Boer Goat
Raising Goats Easy Guide To Raising and Caring for Goats
The Fun of Goats

My Lap Shop Publishers

Plymouth, England

www.mylapshop.com